Tanya G. Guleria

The Most Common Mistakes in Medical Science

Contents:

1. Before We Start...................4

2. The Fifth Way of Excretion of Heavy Metals..................6

3. Stereoscopic Vision Is Not a Privilege Only to Those Who Have Two Eyes in the Same Direction............................8

4. What We Do Wrong By the Implantation of Thoracic Drainage?...........................10

5. What We Do Wrong By the Removing of Thoracic Drainage?..........................12

6. Is Nicotine Really Responsible For The Acute Coronary Disease?............14

7. Psychic disorders may be connected with consumption of beef..............................18

8. Why Osteoporosis is More Common in Countries where Milk Is a Natural Food and Not Where It Is Seldom?..................22

9. The Paradox of Medical Science. 24

Before We Start

As a medical doctor I am often asked a lot of questions. Sometimes I can answer quickly, sometimes I need some time to read, think and analyze. Sometimes the answers come like the apple of Newton, sometimes in my dream like the table of Mendeleev, sometimes it comes on time, sometimes too late to help our patients or beloved ones. Because we doctors are not perfect, our science is also too large and too complicated to understand. But should we give up?

A common mistake that is made in each scientific journey is acceptance. We accept that those who had written our notebooks are always right and their theories are non-questionable. But is that so?

They are also people and they are capable of making mistakes, isn't that so?

In this book I will try to give some examples for the mistakes in medical science and practice, that would make you think and analyze every information that is offered to you. Perhaps this book won't make you a discoverer, but will teach you to think and you would thank me for this lesson.

The Fifth Way of Excretion of Heavy Metals

The first mistake in medical science I met in the books and lectures in hygiene. Our lecturer defined the act of excretion as a process by which metabolic waste is eliminated from an organism. In vertebrates this is primarily carried out by the lungs, kidneys, liver and skin.

He defined also accumulation of heavy metals as a process of absorbing those metals from the environment through the blood stream in the organism, in its tissues and organs with the possibility that those metals at certain circumstances to be released again in the blood stream and cause poisoning.

And he mentioned nails and hair as organs in which heavy metals accumulate.

And that was the point I got perplexed. Could heavy metals be released in the blood stream again after they have been "accumulated" in hair and nails? Why do we call this process accumulation if it responds much better according to the definition to excretion?

So that was the discovery of the fifth way of excretion of heavy metals as a colleague of mine humorously called prophylaxis of heavy metals poisoning through haircut.

Stereoscopic Vision Is Not a Privilege Only to Those Who Have Two Eyes in the Same Direction

Sounds exciting to prove it, but do you really think rabbits and deers have no stereoscopic vision at all?

Stereoscopic vision is a function which occurs if we see one object with more than one point of view. For example two eyes in the same direction. But in our classes in ophthalmology we learnt that our retina changes every second the point with which it sees the objects, because the rod cells and cone cells receive only one impulse of light and then they are exhausted. This means that every object is seen with more points of the retina, So theoretically we should have stereoscopic vision even with one eye. Because the nervous system can analyze the movement of the retina and the eye and the body and so is stereoscopic vision possible even only with one eye and many nervous cells which are stimulated by the rod and the cone cells. Prove? The world is perfectly three-dimensional even if you close one eye even in a completely new situation so your memory cannot be involved.

Of course we do not have the necessary apparatus to register this because they all are on the principle of binocular vision.

What We Do Wrong By the Implantation of Thoracic Drainage?

The most popular technique of implanting thoracic drainage is by Bulau. It is used even if the patient has a pure pneumothorax. For some reason sometimes it is quite ineffective.

Why?

Imagine you try to suck out air through a pipe with many holes which comes from the bottom of a bottle which is halve full with water and you do not use any negative pressure(you do not suck at all). Does it function?

Now you think haematopneumothorax is air and blood in the thorax and the Bulau thoracic drainage comes from underneath the heavy disabled patient who lies all the time on his back. Air is under the sternum or apical and blood is near the ribs dorsocaudal. The idea came to me after seeing the CT scan of a patient with thoracic drainage who died nevertheless after having the Bulau drainage. Of course it was not my patient. And it was on a medical conference.

Naturally you would ask what should we do in such a case? The thoracic drainage by Monaldi is more complicated to be implanted but is according my theory much more effective, because if you put a pipe on the top of a bottle the air under pressure goes by all the physics laws out.

What We Do Wrong By the Removing of Thoracic Drainage?

Another mistake that doctors make is by the removing of thoracic drainage, but it could not be so fatal.

What we do is we command inhale, exhale, press as you have defecation and then we pull out the drainage and close the sack stitches. What is wrong you would ask?

By exhaling we cause the reduction of the negative intrapleural pressure, but by the process of pressing as by defecation the diaphragm goes under to press the abdomen. So the pleura space goes again into higher negative pressure and this may cause repetitive inflow of air in the pleural sack. So you should pull out the thoracic drainage only by the exhaling process, do not make it more complicated.

However this mistake is only a drop into the ocean of imperfections.

Is Nicotine Really Responsible For The Acute Coronary Disease?

All our lives we have been poured with information that cigarette smoking is the reason for acute coronary diseases and peripher arterial atherosclerosis. But is that so?

A lot of scientific works have proved that nicotine has an anti-inflammation effect. This means it reduces the human body immune and autoimmune inflammation. This is the principle of most of the NSAR medicaments which we use so commonly when we have fever, pain and other flue like symptoms.

A lot of scientific works prove that atherosclerosis which is the reason for acute coronary and peripher arterial occlusive diseases has an element of inflammation in it. There were even tries to find some bacteria which could trigger it. Of course all this trials were unsuccessful.

Is it possible that atherosclerosis is an autoimmune disease? Until now no-one has checked such an option. Why? Which antibodies should we blame for it?

It is only an idea but perhaps we should check out the influenza virus cell receptor antibodies. Why?

In the organism influenza virus affects all endothelial cells of blood vessels and bronchial epithelium. This means that we have receptors for influenza virus in our endothelial blood vessel cells. Theoretically if we had antibodies which attack this receptors they would attack blood vessel endothelium, isn't it so?

Why our organism would build such an antibody against its own endothelium?

And let us come back to influenza virus again. It is known that influenza virus affects many species such as pigs and birds. This means that the endothelial cells of those species have similar to human beings influenza virus receptors. How could that affect us?

It is known that our immune system reacts to proteins which contain more than 21 alfa-amino-acids and are somehow different in structure than our own proteins. This means that if the pigs' or birds' receptors for the influenza virus enter our blood stream or lymph stream or organs or body would react to them through the immune system and build antibodies against those influenza virus receptors. What has that to do with atherosclerosis?

We accepted that human and pig and bird cell influenza receptors are similar. Than what would happen if those antibódies falsely react to human influenza virus receptors? - Inflammation of the human blood vessel endothelium. Or isn't it so?

And this is the moment when we come back to atherosclerosis. Have we not proved that it has an inflammatory origin? – Yes, but no-one thought what is the reason or if one thought one was misled.

And let us come back to nicotine. It has anti-inflammatory effect. So perhaps it is protective against atherosclerosis?

No-one has ever researched the way of life of smokers. Most smokers eat meat? or isn't it so? And atherosclerosis is common also in non-smokers. So what is the proof that nicotine causes it? - Actually none.

Psychic disorders may be connected with consumption of beef

A lot of scientific trials prove that psychic disorders like schizophrenia, autism, dementia, Alzheimer, Parkinson syndrome have an inflammatory character. Some of them are proven to be connected with irritable bowel syndrome but the connection is until now unclear. Is it the psychic disorder that causes the irritable bowel or just the opposite. So what would you say?

In my opinion the irritable bowel syndrome provides an inflammation process in the large intestines that causes minimal injuries in the bowel. So protein molecules from the food can enter lymph stream and blood stream and cause an immune reaction to them by building antibodies. If those proteins are similar to human nerve cell proteins this may cause that those antibodies react also falsely with human nerve cell proteins and cause their demolition through the immune system.

Any proof?

Jacobs-Kreuzfeld disease is a parallel disease in humans and bovines. It is caused by a protein molecule which can connect itself with a receptor of the nerve cell and enter into the nerve cell and replicate itself through its genetic system and is called prion. The fact that it is common in humans and bovines proves that the prion receptor in humans and cows is common. This means that the reaction to the bovine prion receptor by the human immune system causes production of antibodies which react falsely with the human prion receptor.

Thus psychic disorders are caused not only by the prion (by Jacobs Kreuzfeld disease) but also through the immune reaction of the human organism against the nerve prion receptor in beef and the false recognition of the human nerve receptor by the antibodies produced to react to the bovine prion receptor. In human brain this autoimmune reaction causes destruction of neurons and the above mentioned diseases.

Which of the above mentioned diseases would develop the person depends on against which receptor in brain is the autoimmune reaction and where is it found. For example the Parkinson syndrome is caused by destruction of substantia nigra in brain stem, Alzheimer by destruction of neurons in the frontal part of the hemispheres, etc.

In conclusion psychic disorders are not only inflammatory but also autoimmune. Through injuries in the intestinal wall in the lymph stream enter foreign protein molecules that cause an immune reaction and producing antibodies. Those antibodies could react falsely with human brain cells receptors which are similar to those antigens.

Sounds logical, or?

Why Osteoporosis is More Common in Countries where Milk Is a Natural Food and Not Where It Is Seldom?

The so called calcium sensing receptor is found in the bone cells. It regulates the bone cells metabolism. Targeting the bone Calcium sensing receptors using a bone-seeking Calcium sensing receptor agonist offers a potential mean to modulate bone cell metabolism. The development of drugs that preferentially target the Calcium sensor receptor and possibly other calcium-sensing receptors in bone cells may thus be helpful for the treatment of osteoporosis.

So if we assume that in our body exist antibodies which attack this receptor this may be the reason of osteoporosis, or?

How could the production of those antibodies be caused is not so far from mind if you have carefully read the previous articles.

Is osteoporosis an autoimmune reaction to Calcium-sensing receptors? - Why not if we follow our new principles.

So let us summarize: the intake of similar Calcium sensing receptors from meat and milk can trigger the production of antibodies which falsely attack the human calcium sensing receptor thus damaging the intake of calcium in the cell and the production of carbonated hydroxyapatite which is the main bone mineral substance. Perhaps this explanation is too complicated, but it is enough to enlighten the paradox in the connection of milk products consumption and osteoporosis.

This also explains why biphosphonates such as alendronic acid can increase bone density, but do not affect the bone fragility at all.

The Paradox of Medical Science

The paradox of medical science nowadays is that it explains all diseases with imperfection of metabolism as if we have been born to get sick and take tablets. Human organism is a product of hundred thousands of years of evolution. So if we accept we are so imperfect how could we survive for so long?

Nature is a perfectionist, it demolishes everything that is useless and cannot multiply. Diseases are the way the natural selection functions. And it may be brutal but natural selection perhaps tells us we should think more about our way of life if we want to be healthy. It does not work for the medical firms so that they could get richer from human suffering. If this small book has been interesting for you, read "The Theory of Autoimmunity" and your mind would be blown.

Just remember: Knowledge is power and all powers are afraid of knowledge.

www.ingramcontent.com/pod-product-compliance
Lightning Source LLC
Chambersburg PA
CBHW032312240526
45464CB00023BA/3001

Spirit 5
The Beginning
INTRODUCTION

I have created four super human characters the first is Benjamin and he is the spirit five, an assassin from the world that looks over the planet earth. How I created him, I guess it was through the thought though my mind the idea was that he was to eliminate seven extremely important people who had miss used their judgement and powers governing the planet earth they were to be punished. As every superhero has a story there is a good part and a bad part one minute he would be doing things for the good and other times he would be doing thing for the bad. The hero in this story is all bad in his case the bad guys win and there is a curse to go with it as Benjamin must live with the five super powers that process him. In this case it is the same, but there is a story to it.

I do not know how I came about it, one minute I was sitting there on my stool writing in the dark the next minute I had created him Benjamin. Benjamin is the spirit. On top of this I had some more characters that I had created. I decided at the time that the story needed a bit of help, so I decided to add a couple of futuristic coppers called the oxygen and the hitman and gave them a car called the cool one, after the number plate which was private on their car, Benjamin is close to it as it is close to the public. They do not like it, there must be bad guys in the story and there both it. not forgetting the real master, the silhouette, a sassy cool individual and killer that brings Benjamin down a good looking cool adversary that has the power to bring the Benjamin down he that bad guy in the story. Who will win, who knows yet have a read.

As I continue, Benjamin knows that there is something going on in planet earth and that's the only reason that he is there. Benjamin has some help from his friends a robot that we call a robot some of the time and other time's we call him mar arty and a couple of crazy sun flowers called the flowers to guide him.

Preface

Benjamin knows that there is something wrong on the planet earth the story go's he is busy moving to a new house he is upstairs in his attic. As he clears the boxes in his attic he stumbles getting ready to move he stubbles across an old tin at first, he ignores it but the feeling that the tin gave him drew him back to it, so he puts it aside for another time except he is drawn to it more the more he tries to disregard the thought the more his mind thinks about it. he is extremely drawn to it. as the next few days past looking at the box he decides to open it and when he doe's he finds a magic badge. This badge is extremely special and once it is on you it cannot be removed from the clothing and will slowly become part of the body. Benjamin does not know this at first, Benjamin decides to fly to Britain to a professor to find the meaning of the badge and wants to know what exactly what it's purpose.